Scrumptious Overnight Oats

Irresistible healthy but flavourful Recipes To start your Day.

By

Marisela Alonso

Table of contents

Introduction

Rise and shine, breakfast connoisseurs! Have you ever found yourself in a morning rut, frantically looking for a quick, nutritious meal that is more intriguing than plain toast? Welcome to your new morning BFF, "scrumptious Overnight Oats: irresistible healthy but flavorful Recipes to Start Your Day!"

Let's face it: before coffee, mornings may be a little like solving a Rubik's Cube. But don't worry, since this book is your secret to morning bliss!

Consider this: delicious overnight oats dishes that will make your taste senses sing! This book has more variety than your favorite pizza shop, with everything from traditional tastes to crazy fruity blends, nutty creations to desserts in a bowl.

Whether you're a busy bee, a health freak, or just weary of breakfast dullness, these dishes are here to help. They're as simple to make as your favorite burger and as delicious as a weekend brunch with friends.

So be ready to change your dreary morning ritual. Grab a spoon, join the overnight oats train, and turn breakfast into your favorite time of the day!

Chapter 1

Getting Started with Overnight Oats

What exactly is overnight oats?

Overnight oats are just oats that have been allowed to refrigerate overnight rather than cooked in the morning, making them ideal for a quick, satisfying, and healthy breakfast. Overnight oats are a no-cook technique of cooking oatmeal that requires soaking oats in liquid overnight in the refrigerator, such as milk, juice, or yogurt. Overnight, the oats absorb the liquid and soften, resulting in a ready-to-eat breakfast in the morning. This method does not need heating; instead, the soaking process softens and the oats. It's a handy and adaptable method to have a healthy breakfast, since different components such as fruits, nuts, seeds, sweeteners, or flavorings may be added to produce a variety of tastes and textures. Overnight oats are a popular option for hectic mornings due to their ease, variety, and ability to be made ahead of time.

Overnight oats are distinct in that their molecular make-up has not been altered by heat. As a consequence, the oatmeal becomes creamier and has slowly and profoundly absorbed the flavors of anything you've combined it with.

Of course, there are occasions when you just want the comfort of a cooked breakfast. But when you know you'll need something fast and tasty that's going to set your day off to a wonderful start, it may be time to try soaking some oats!.

Benefits of Overnight Oats

Breakfast kings and queens! Overnight oats are the ideal breakfast shortcut.
Consider this: you combine oats with your favorite milk or yogurt, put it in the fridge overnight, and voila! You've got a delicious, no-cook breakfast ready to go in the morning.

What's the greatest part? You're in charge! Do you want to add some fruits, nuts, or honey? You do what you want! Oh, and these oats are the best at keeping you satisfied and healthy. They're high in fiber, which helps keep hunger at bay and your stomach satisfied. Plus, they're very quick to grab and go, making them ideal for those hectic mornings!

So, if you're looking for easy, substantial breakfasts, oats are a terrific source of protein and fiber, as well as other vitamins and minerals like calcium, manganese, and phosphorus, among other things.
Below is a more extensive breakdown of some of the advantages of overnight oats.

1. Ease of preparation: Prepare them the night before for a hassle-free, ready-to-eat breakfast in the morning.

2. Time-saving: There is no need to cook; just soak oats overnight and have a quick meal.

3. Customizable: Create your own flavor combinations using fruits, nuts, seeds, or sweeteners.

4. Nutritious: High in fiber, vitamins, and minerals, it promotes a balanced diet and aids digestion.

5. Filling: Their high fiber content keeps you fuller for longer, helping to regulate appetite throughout the morning.

6. Gut Health: Its fiber content promotes a pleasant and balanced digestive system by supporting a healthy gut.

7. Portable: It's easy to take for on-the-go breakfast, making it excellent for hectic mornings or as a packed meal choice.

8. Versatile: Adaptable to a variety of nutritional demands, such as vegan, gluten-free, or high-protein, while catering to a variety of lifestyles.

9. Shelf life: Yes, you may cook overnight oats and keep them in the refrigerator for up to 5 days.

Essential Ingredients and Tools Required

1. Oats: Many overnight oats experts will tell you that rolled oats (also known as old-fashioned oats) are the only way to proceed. Rolled oats are entire oat groats that have been rolled flat. Because this is their sole processing, they are more nutritious than other forms of oats. Rolled oats retain some bite and do not become as mushy or gloopy as other varieties of oats. That's why they're popular, but maybe a softer consistency is just what you're looking for?

If this is the case, try either regular or quick oats. Regular oats have been steamed and ground, but the processing is still modest, giving them a healthy breakfast alternative that is still a touch chunky in the morning. Quick oats, as the name implies, are finely ground oats that cook rapidly. They become incredibly soft and simple to digest after being soaked overnight.

It's worth noting that quick oats are also known as instant oats. These are not the same as quick oatmeal. Quick oatmeal or quick porridge is a highly processed foodstuff that yields soupy (and unhealthy) overnight oats. These should be avoided.

2. Liquid: Milk (dairy or nondairy, such as almond, soy, oat, or coconut milk) or yogurt is used to refrigerate the oats. This is critical since it is what you refrigerate your oats in to get that creamy texture. Yummy yummy!

3. Sweetener: This is Optional but commonly used for added flavor and sweetness - honey, maple syrup, agave nectar, or even mashed ripe bananas are added as sweeteners

4. Mix-ins/ Flavorings: this is also optional but necessary.Mix-ins are the ingredients you should stir into your oats and milk to let stand overnight.We have Vanilla extract, cinnamon, coffee,pumpkin spice mix, Chia spice mix and other spices to enhance taste and smell.

5. Toppings: These are the ingredients you should chuck onto your overnight oats right before eating.
Fruits (fresh or dried), nuts, seeds (chia, flaxseed), shredded coconut, or peanut butter, chocolate chips,toasted almonds Broken biscuits/cookies for texture and added nutrients.

Tools:

1. Container: Mason jars or any airtight container with a lid for preparing and storing the oats.

2. Measuring Cups/Spoons: To accurately measure oats, liquids, sweeteners, and other ingredients.

3. Stirring Utensil: A spoon or spatula for mixing the ingredients thoroughly.

4. Refrigerator: Access to a fridge for overnight soaking and storage of the oats.

These ingredients and tools make preparing overnight oats a walk in the park, allowing for ease of preparation ahead of time.

Chapter 2

Classic Overnight oats recipes

Basic Vanilla Overnight Oats recipe

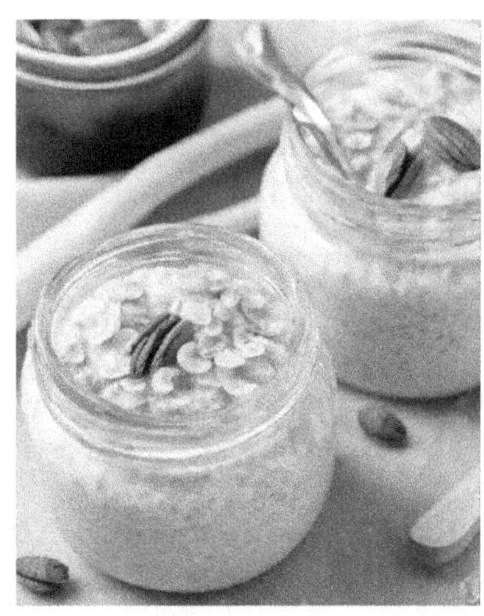

Prep Time: 5 minutes

Serving: just 1 serving

Ingredients:
- 1/2 cup rolled oats (old-fashioned oats)
- 1/2 cup milk (dairy or non-dairy)
- 1 tablespoon honey or maple syrup (optional)
- 1/2 teaspoon vanilla extract
- Pinch of salt (optional)

Method:
1. Combine Ingredients: In a jar or container with a lid, add rolled oats, milk, honey or maple syrup (if using), vanilla extract, and a pinch of salt if desired.

2. Mix Well:Stir all the ingredients until thoroughly combined.

3. Refrigerate:Seal the jar/container with a lid and place it in the refrigerator. Let it refrigerate overnight or for at least 4-5 hours.

4. Serve: The next morning, give the oats a good stir. If desired, add additional milk to adjust consistency.

5. Enjoy: Your delicious and creamy Basic Vanilla Overnight Oats are ready to fuel your morning!

Adjust sweetness or consistency by adding more or less sweetener or milk according to personal taste preferences.

Berry Blast Overnight Oats recipe

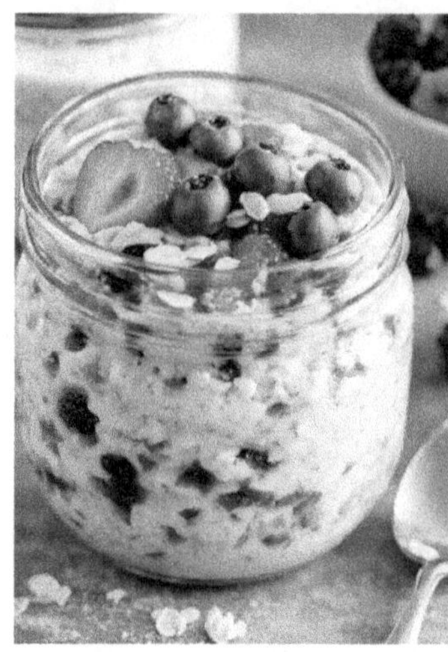

Prep Time: 5 minutes

Serving: just 1 serving

Ingredients:
- 1/2 cup rolled oats (old-fashioned oats)
- 1/2 cup milk (dairy or non-dairy)
- 1/4 cup plain yogurt
- 1 tablespoon honey or maple syrup (optional, depending on sweetness preference)
- 1/2 teaspoon vanilla extract
- 1/2 cup mixed berries (strawberries, blueberries, raspberries)
- A handful of sliced strawberries for topping (optional)
- A few extra berries for garnish (optional)

Method:

1. Combine Ingredients: In a jar or container with a lid, add rolled oats, milk, plain yogurt, honey or maple syrup (if using), vanilla extract, and mixed berries.

2. Mix Well: Stir all the ingredients until thoroughly combined.

3. Refrigerate: Seal the jar/container with a lid and place it in the refrigerator. Allow it to refrigerate overnight or for at least 4 hours.

4. Serve:The next morning, give the oats a good stir. If desired, add more milk for preferred consistency. Top with sliced strawberries and extra berries for garnish.

5. Enjoy: Your Classic Berry Blast Overnight Oats are ready to add a burst of fruity flavor to your morning routine!

This recipe creates a single serving of delicious berry-infused overnight oats. Feel free to adjust sweetness or add more berries according to your taste.

Chocolate Peanut Butter Delight Recipe

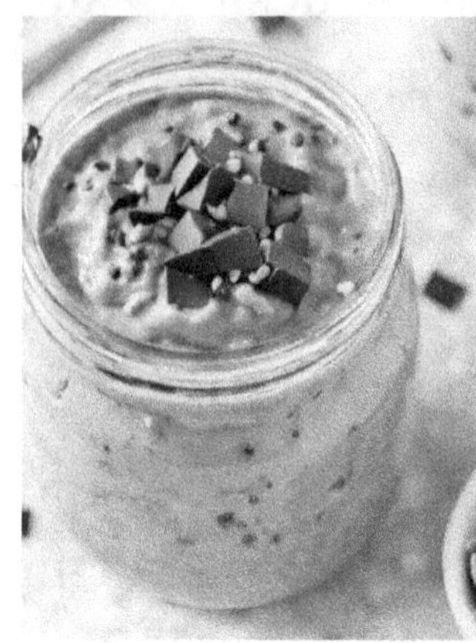

Prep Time: 5 minutes

Serving: just 1 serving

Ingredients:
- 1/2 cup rolled oats (old-fashioned oats)
- 1/2 cup milk (dairy or non-dairy)
- 1 tablespoon cocoa powder
- 1 tablespoon peanut butter (creamy or crunchy)
- 1 tablespoon honey or maple syrup (optional, for sweetness)
- 1/2 teaspoon vanilla extract
- A pinch of salt (optional)
- Chopped peanuts or mini chocolate chips for topping (optional)

Method:

1. In a jar or container, combine rolled oats, milk, cocoa powder, peanut butter, honey or maple syrup, vanilla extract, and a pinch of salt. Stir well until thoroughly mixed.

2. Seal the jar or container and place it in the refrigerator. Let it refrigerate overnight or for at least 4-5 hours.

3. The next morning, give the oats a good stir. Add more milk if desired for preferred consistency.

4. Top with chopped peanuts or mini chocolate chips if you like.

5. Enjoy your delicious Chocolate Peanut Butter Delight Overnight Oat. Adjust ingredients to suit your taste preferences and indulge in this delightful chocolatey and nutty combination.

Cinnamon Apple Pie Overnight Oats recipe

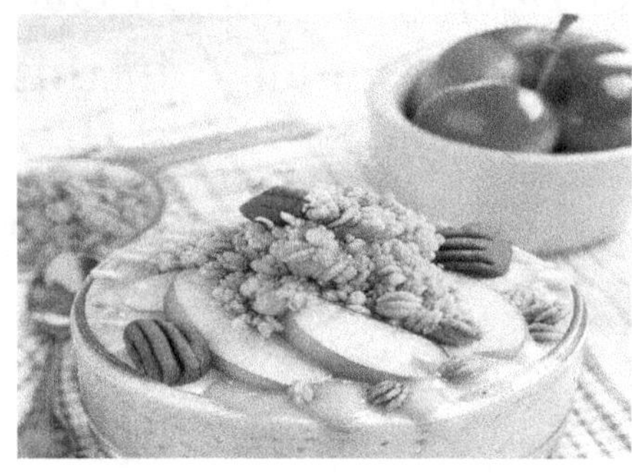

Prep Time: 5 minutes

Serving: just 1 serving

Ingredients:
- 1/2 cup rolled oats (old-fashioned oats)
- 1/2 cup milk (dairy or non-dairy)
- 1/2 cup unsweetened applesauce
- 1 tablespoon maple syrup or honey
- 1/2 teaspoon ground cinnamon
- 1/4 teaspoon ground nutmeg (optional)
- 1/2 teaspoon vanilla extract
- Chopped apple pieces for topping (optional)
- Granola or chopped nuts for topping (optional)

Method:

1. In a jar or container, combine rolled oats, milk, unsweetened applesauce, maple syrup or honey, ground cinnamon, ground nutmeg (if using), and vanilla extract. Mix well until thoroughly combined.

2. Seal the jar or container and place it in the refrigerator. Allow it to refrigerate overnight or for at least 4 hours.

3. The next morning, give the oats a good stir. If needed, add more milk for desired consistency.

4. Top with chopped apple pieces, granola, or chopped nuts for extra texture and flavor.

5. Enjoy your delightful Cinnamon Apple Pie Overnight Oats! This recipe brings the comforting flavors of apple pie into a healthy breakfast, perfect for satisfying your morning cravings. Adjust sweetness or spices according to your taste preferences.

Banana Nut Bliss Overnight Oat Recipe

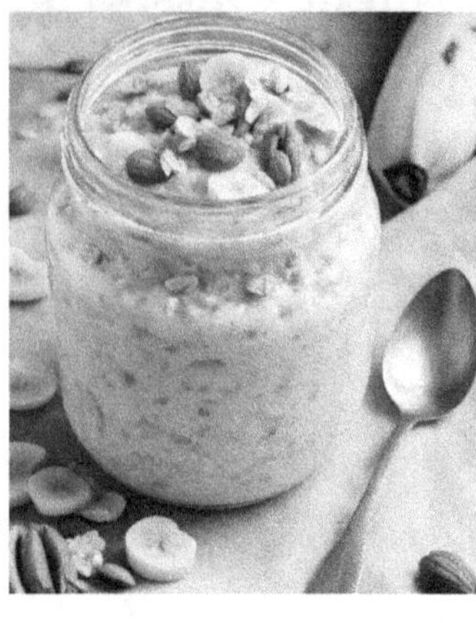

Prep Time: 5 minutes

Serving: just 1 serving

Ingredients:
- 1/2 cup rolled oats (old-fashioned oats)
- 1/2 cup milk (dairy or non-dairy)
- 1 ripe banana, mashed
- 1 tablespoon honey or maple syrup
- 1/4 teaspoon ground cinnamon
- 2 tablespoons chopped nuts (walnuts, almonds, pecans, etc.)
- A few slices of banana for topping (optional)

Method:

1. In a jar or container, combine rolled oats, milk, mashed ripe banana, honey or maple syrup, ground cinnamon, and chopped nuts. Stir well to ensure everything is thoroughly mixed.

2. Seal the jar or container and place it in the refrigerator. Allow it to refrigerate overnight or for at least 4 hours.

3. The next morning, give the oats a good stir. If needed, add more milk for desired consistency.

4. Top with a few slices of banana for garnish or extra sweetness if you'd like.

5. Enjoy your creamy and nutty Banana Nut Bliss Overnight Oats! This recipe combines the natural sweetness of bananas with the crunch of nuts, creating a delightful breakfast treat. Feel free to adjust sweetness or add more nuts for your preferred taste and texture.

Chapter 3: Fruity Creations

Mango Tango Overnight Oats recipe

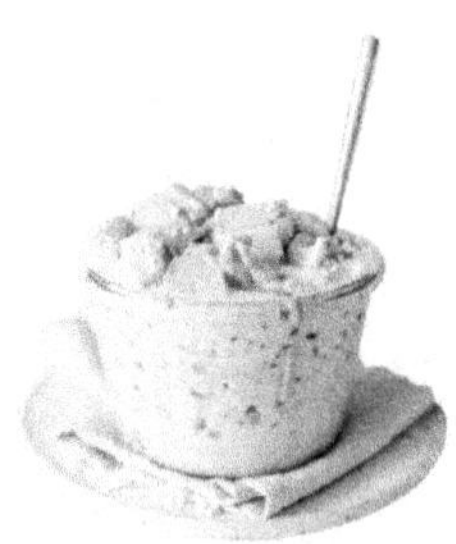

Prep Time: 5 minutes

Serving: just 1 serving

Ingredients:
- 1/2 cup rolled oats (old-fashioned oats)
- 1/2 cup milk (dairy or non-dairy)
- 1/2 cup diced ripe mango
- 1 tablespoon honey or maple syrup (optional, based on sweetness preference)
- 1/4 teaspoon vanilla extract
- A pinch of ground ginger (optional, for a spicy kick)
- Sliced mango or shredded coconut for topping (optional)

Method:

1. In a jar or container, combine rolled oats, milk, diced ripe mango, honey or maple syrup (if desired), vanilla extract, and a pinch of ground ginger if using. Mix well until all ingredients are thoroughly combined.

2. Seal the jar or container and place it in the refrigerator. Allow it to refrigerate overnight or for a minimum of 4 hours.

3. The next morning, stir the oats well. If the consistency is too thick, add a splash of milk and mix.

4. Top your Mango Tango Overnight Oats with additional sliced mango or shredded coconut for an extra tropical touch if desired.

5. Enjoy your delightful and fruity Mango Tango Overnight Oats! This recipe brings the refreshing taste of mangoes into your breakfast, providing a burst of tropical flavors to kickstart your day. Adjust sweetness or spice level to suit your taste preferences.

Tropical Pineapple Paradise Overnight Oat recipe

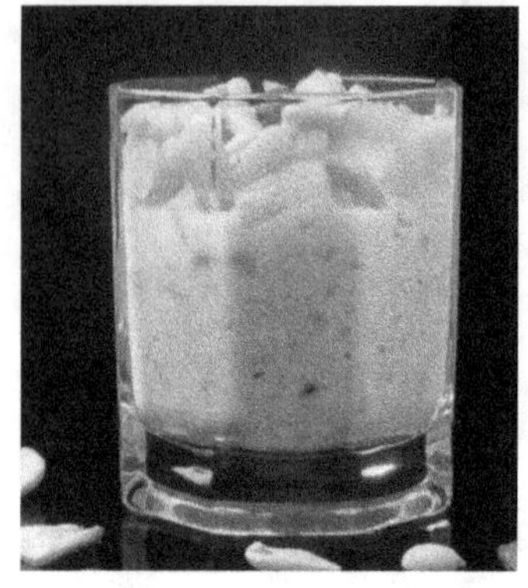

Prep Time: 5 minutes

Serving: 1 serving

Ingredients:
- 1/2 cup rolled oats (old-fashioned oats)
- 1/2 cup milk (dairy or non-dairy)
- 1/2 cup diced fresh pineapple
- 2 tablespoons unsweetened shredded coconut
- 1 tablespoon honey or maple syrup (optional, for added sweetness)
- 1/4 teaspoon vanilla extract
- A sprinkle of chopped nuts (macadamia, almonds, or cashews) for topping (optional)

Method:

1. In a jar or container, combine rolled oats, milk, diced fresh pineapple, unsweetened shredded coconut, honey or maple syrup (if using), and vanilla extract. Stir well to thoroughly mix all ingredients.

2. Seal the jar or container and place it in the refrigerator. Let it refrigerate overnight or for at least 4 hours.

3. The next morning, give the oats a good stir. If the mixture is too thick, add a splash of milk and mix well.

4. Top your Tropical Pineapple Paradise Overnight Oats with a sprinkle of chopped nuts for added crunch and flavor if desired.

5. Enjoy the tropical goodness of your Pineapple Paradise Overnight Oats! This recipe transports you to a tropical paradise with the refreshing taste of pineapple and coconut.

Mixed Berry Medley Overnight Oat recipe

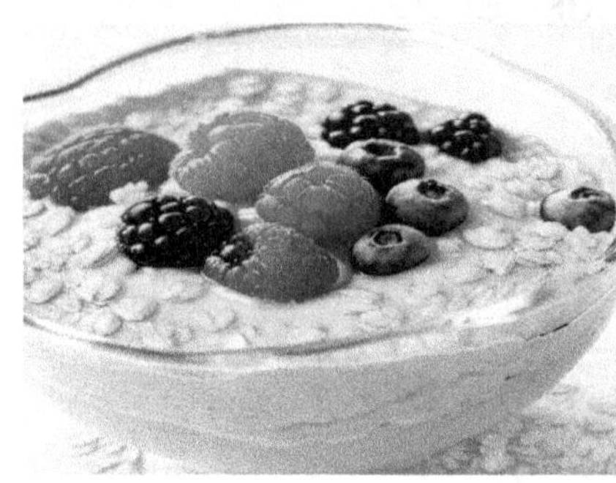

Prep Time: 5 minutes

Serving: 1 serving

Ingredients:
- 1/2 cup rolled oats (old-fashioned oats)
- 1/2 cup milk (dairy or non-dairy)
- 1/2 cup mixed berries (strawberries, blueberries, raspberries)
- 1 tablespoon honey or maple syrup (optional, for sweetness)
- 1/4 teaspoon vanilla extract
- A handful of mixed berries for topping (optional)

Method:

1. In a jar or container, combine rolled oats, milk, mixed berries, honey or maple syrup (if desired), and vanilla extract. Stir well to ensure all ingredients are evenly mixed.

2. Seal the jar or container and place it in the refrigerator. Allow it to refrigerate overnight or for at least 4 hours.

3. The next morning, give the oats a good stir. If the consistency is too thick, add a splash of milk and mix well.

4. Top your Mixed Berry Medley Overnight Oats with an extra handful of mixed berries for a burst of freshness and flavor if desired.

5. Enjoy your Mixed Berry Medley Overnight Oats! This recipe brings the vibrant and sweet taste of assorted berries into your breakfast, creating a delightful and colorful morning treat. Adjust sweetness or add more berries according to your taste preferences.

Pomegranate Power Oats recipe

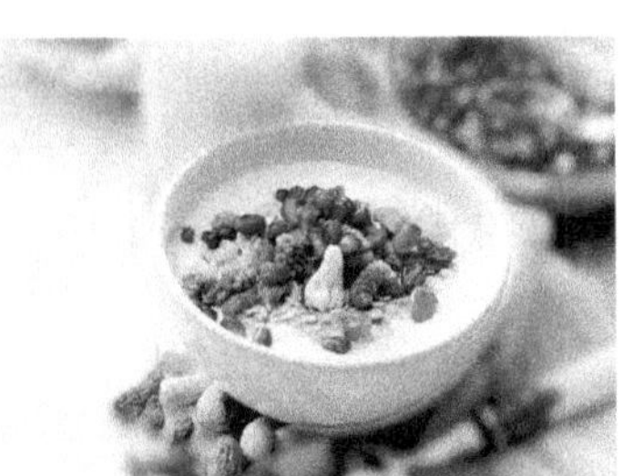

Prep Time: 5 minutes

Serving: just 1 **serving**

Ingredients:
- 1/2 cup rolled oats (old-fashioned oats)
- 1/2 cup milk (dairy or non-dairy)
- 1/4 cup pomegranate arils (seeds)
- 1 tablespoon honey or maple syrup (optional, for sweetness)
- 1/4 teaspoon vanilla extract
- A sprinkle of chia seeds or chopped nuts for topping (optional)

Method:

1. In a jar or container, combine rolled oats, milk, pomegranate arils, honey or maple syrup (if using), and vanilla extract. Mix well to ensure all ingredients are thoroughly combined.

2. Seal the jar or container and place it in the refrigerator. Allow it to refrigerate overnight or for a minimum of 4 hours.

3. The next morning, give the oats a good stir. If the mixture is too thick, add a little more milk and mix well.

4. Top your Pomegranate Power Overnight Oats with a sprinkle of chia seeds or chopped nuts for added texture and nutritional value if desired.

5. Enjoy the vibrant and nutritious Pomegranate Power Overnight Oats! This recipe introduces the sweet and tangy taste of pomegranate arils into your breakfast, providing a refreshing and antioxidant-rich morning boost. Adjust sweetness or add more toppings according to your liking.

Citrus Sunrise Overnight Oats recipe

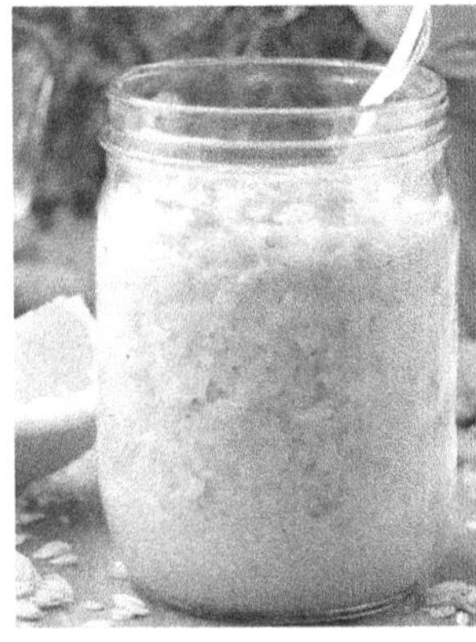

Prep Time: 5 minutes

Serving: 1

Ingredients:
- 1/2 cup rolled oats (old-fashioned oats)
- 1/2 cup orange juice (freshly squeezed or store-bought)
- Zest of 1 orange (optional, for extra citrus flavor)
- 1 tablespoon honey or maple syrup (optional, for sweetness)
- 1/4 teaspoon vanilla extract
- Slices of orange for topping (optional)

Method:
1. In a jar or container, combine rolled oats, orange juice, orange zest (if using), honey or maple syrup (if desired), and vanilla extract. Stir well to ensure all ingredients are thoroughly mixed.

2. Seal the jar or container and place it in the refrigerator. Allow it to refrigerate overnight or for a minimum of 4 hours.

3. The next morning, stir the oats well. If the consistency is too thick, add a splash of orange juice and mix until you achieve your desired consistency.

4. Top your Citrus Sunrise Overnight Oats with slices of orange for a zesty and refreshing topping if desired.

5. Enjoy the refreshing burst of citrus flavor in your Citrus Sunrise Overnight Oats! This recipe brings the tangy and invigorating taste of oranges into your breakfast, providing a delightful and vitamin-packed start to your day. Adjust sweetness or add more orange zest according to your taste preferences.

Chapter 4: Nutty and Seedy Combinations

Almond Joy Overnight Oats recipe

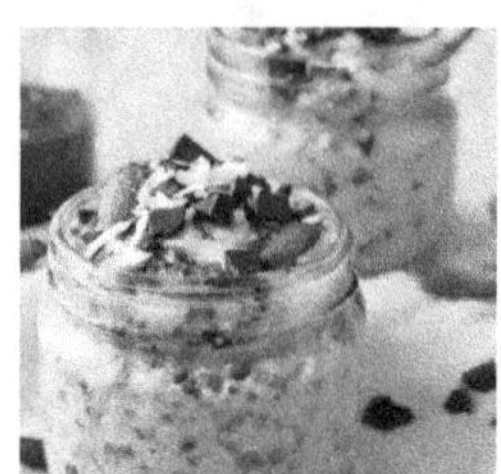

Prep Time: 5 minutes

Serving: 1

Ingredients:
- 1/2 cup rolled oats (old-fashioned oats)
- 1/2 cup almond milk (or any milk of your choice)
- 2 tablespoons shredded coconut (unsweetened)
- 1 tablespoon cocoa powder
- 1 tablespoon honey or maple syrup (optional, for sweetness)
- 1 tablespoon chopped almonds
- 1 tablespoon mini chocolate chips (optional, for extra taste)
- A sprinkle of additional shredded coconut for topping (optional)

Method:

1. In a jar or container, combine rolled oats, almond milk, shredded coconut, cocoa powder, honey or maple syrup (if using), chopped almonds, and mini chocolate chips if desired. Mix well until all ingredients are evenly combined.

2. Seal the jar or container and place it in the refrigerator. Let it refrigerate overnight or for at least 4 hours.

3. The next morning, give the oats a good stir. If the mixture is too thick, add a splash of almond milk and mix well.

4. Top your Almond Joy Overnight Oats with a sprinkle of shredded coconut for an extra coconutty crunch if desired.

5. Enjoy the delightful flavors of Almond Joy in your breakfast! This recipe combines the richness of chocolate and coconut with the nutty goodness of almonds, making it a delicious and satisfying morning treat. Adjust sweetness or add more toppings to suit your taste preferences.

Crunchy Cashew Caramel Overnight Oat recipe

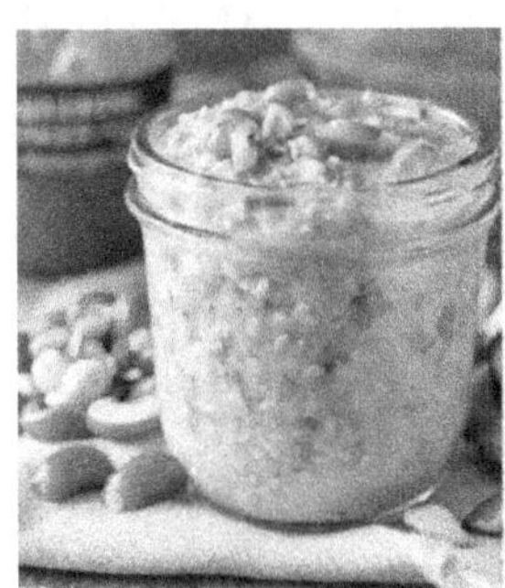

Prep Time: 5 minutes

Serving: 1

Ingredients:
- 1/2 cup rolled oats (old-fashioned oats)
- 1/2 cup milk (dairy or non-dairy)
- 1 tablespoon caramel sauce (store-bought or homemade)
- 2 tablespoons chopped cashews
- 1 tablespoon honey or maple syrup (optional, for added sweetness)
- A pinch of salt (optional)
- Additional chopped cashews for topping (optional, for extra crunch)

Method:

1. In a jar or container, combine rolled oats, milk, caramel sauce, chopped cashews, honey or maple syrup (if using), and a pinch of salt if desired. Stir well to ensure all ingredients are thoroughly mixed.

2. Seal the jar or container and place it in the refrigerator. Allow it to refrigerate overnight or for a minimum of 4 hours.

3. The next morning, stir the oats well. If the consistency is too thick, add a splash of milk and mix until you achieve your desired consistency.

4. Top your Crunchy Cashew Caramel Overnight Oats with additional chopped cashews for an extra crunch if desired.

5. Enjoy the delightful Crunchy Cashew Caramel flavor in your breakfast! This recipe combines the sweet taste of caramel with the nutty crunch of cashews, creating a tasty and satisfying morning meal. Adjust sweetness or add more toppings according to your preference.

Chia Seed Pudding Overnight Oats recipe

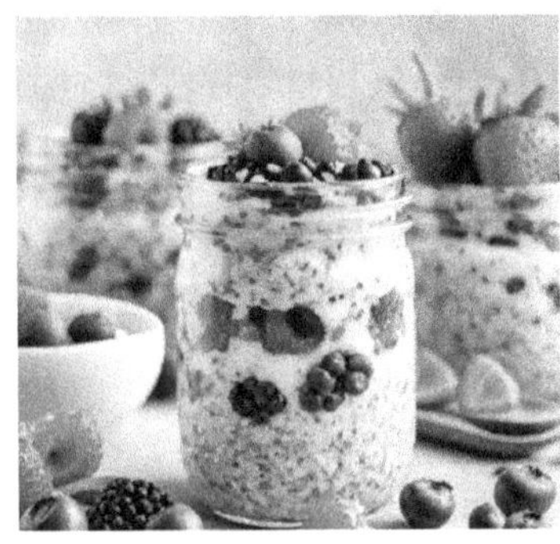

Prep Time: 5 minutes (plus soaking time)

Serving: 1

Ingredients:
- 1/4 cup chia seeds
- 1/2 cup rolled oats (old-fashioned oats)
- 1 cup milk (dairy or non-dairy)
- 1 tablespoon honey or maple syrup (optional, for sweetness)
- 1/2 teaspoon vanilla extract
- Fresh fruit or berries for topping (optional)

Method:

1. In a bowl or jar, combine chia seeds, rolled oats, milk, honey or maple syrup (if using), and vanilla extract. Mix well to ensure all ingredients are thoroughly combined.

2. Seal the bowl or jar and place it in the refrigerator. Let it refrigerate overnight or for a minimum of 5 hours. The mixture will thicken as the chia seeds absorb the liquid.

3. The next morning, stir the chia seed pudding oats thoroughly. If it's too thick, add milk and mix well to reach your preferred consistency.

4. Top your Chia Seed Pudding Overnight Oats with fresh fruit or berries for a burst of flavor and added freshness if desired.

5. Enjoy the combined goodness of chia seed pudding and oats! This recipe offers a delightful blend of creamy pudding-like texture from chia seeds and the heartiness of oats. Adjust sweetness or add toppings to match your taste preferences.

Walnut Maple Overnight Oats

Recipe

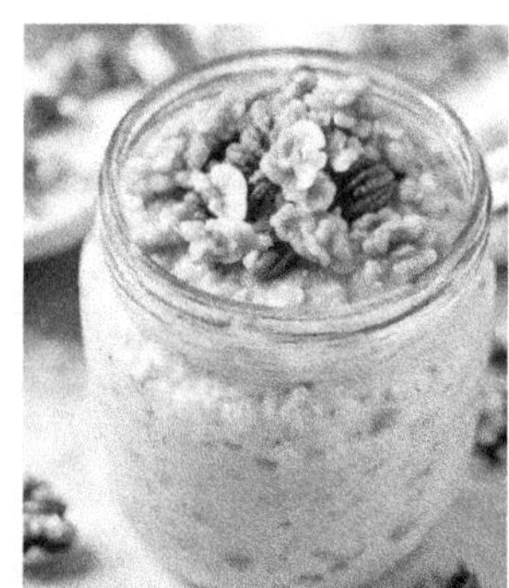

Prep Time: 5 minutes

Serving: 1

Ingredients:
- 1/2 cup rolled oats (old-fashioned oats)
- 1/2 cup milk (dairy or non-dairy)
- 2 tablespoons chopped walnuts
- 1 tablespoon maple syrup
- A sprinkle of cinnamon (optional)
- Additional chopped walnuts for topping (optional)

Method:

1. In a jar or container, combine rolled oats, milk, chopped walnuts, maple syrup, and a sprinkle of cinnamon if desired. Mix well to ensure all ingredients are thoroughly combined.

2. Seal the jar or container and place it in the refrigerator. Allow it to refrigerate overnight or for a minimum of 4 hours.

3. The next morning, stir the oats thoroughly. If the mixture is too thick, add a splash of milk and mix well to achieve your desired consistency.

4. Top your Walnut Maple Overnight Oats with additional chopped walnuts for an extra nutty crunch if desired.

5. Enjoy the delightful blend of nutty walnuts and sweet maple syrup in your breakfast! This recipe combines the rich flavor of walnuts with the sweetness of maple for a comforting and hearty breakfast. Adjust sweetness or add more toppings according to your taste.

Sunflower Seed Honey Overnight Oats recipe

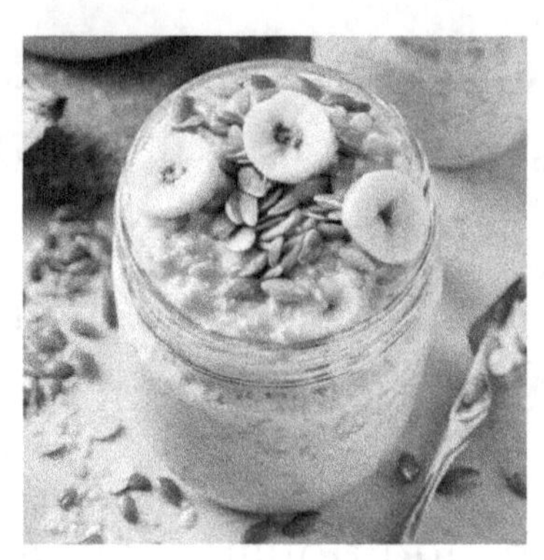

Sunflower seeds can bring several benefits and a unique taste to your overnight oats. Sunflower seeds can provide a nutrient-packed, textural, and flavorful addition to your overnight oats, elevating both the nutritional content and eating experience.

Prep Time: 5 minutes

Serving: 1

Ingredients:
- 1/2 cup rolled oats (old-fashioned oats)
- 1/2 cup milk (dairy or non-dairy)
- 2 tablespoons sunflower seeds
- 1 tablespoon honey
- A pinch of salt (optional)
- Sliced bananas or berries for topping (optional)

Method:

1. In a jar or container, combine rolled oats, milk, sunflower seeds, honey, and a pinch of salt if desired. Stir well to ensure all ingredients are thoroughly mixed.

2. Seal the jar or container and place it in the refrigerator. Allow it to refrigerate overnight or for at least 4 hours.

3. The next morning, stir the oats thoroughly. If the mixture is too thick, add a splash of milk and mix well to reach your desired consistency.

4. Top your Sunflower Seed Honey Overnight Oats with sliced bananas or berries for a fruity addition if desired.

Chapter 5

Dessert-Inspired Overnight Oats Recipes

Cookies and Cream Dream Overnight Oats recipe

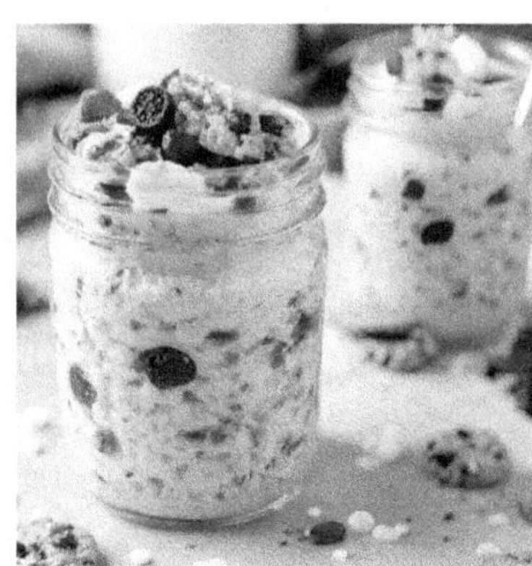

Prep Time: 5 minutes

Serving: 1

Ingredients:
- 1/2 cup rolled oats (old-fashioned oats)
- 1/2 cup milk (dairy or non-dairy)
- 2 chocolate sandwich cookies (like Oreo), crushed
- 1 tablespoon honey or maple syrup (optional, for sweetness)
- 1/4 teaspoon vanilla extract
- Additional cookie crumbs for topping (optional)

Method:

1. In a jar or container, combine rolled oats, milk, crushed chocolate sandwich cookies, honey or maple syrup (if using), and vanilla extract. Mix well to ensure all ingredients are thoroughly combined.

2. Seal the jar or container and place it in the refrigerator. Allow it to refrigerate overnight or for a minimum of 4 hours.

3. The next morning, stir the oats thoroughly. If the mixture is too thick, add a splash of milk and mix well to reach your desired consistency.

4. Top your Cookies and Cream Dream Overnight Oats with additional cookie crumbs for an extra cookie crunch if desired.

5. Enjoy the unique flavor of cookies and cream in your breakfast! This recipe combines the classic taste of chocolate sandwich cookies with creamy oats for a delicious and slightly decadent morning treat. Adjust sweetness or add more toppings according to your preference.

Carrot Cake Overnight Oats recipe

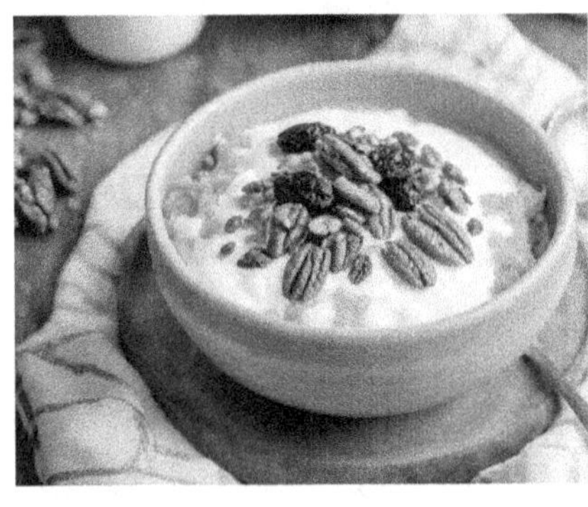

This is just a simple mix of oats, grated carrots, nuts, spices, and a touch of sweetness. Prep it the night before, wake up to a tasty breakfast that's ready to enjoy. Give it a shot for a unique twist on your morning oats!

Prep Time: 5 minutes

Serving: 1

Ingredients:
- 1/2 cup rolled oats (old-fashioned oats)

- 1/2 cup milk (dairy or non-dairy)
- 1/4 cup grated carrots
- 2 tablespoons chopped walnuts or pecans
- 1 tablespoon raisins or chopped dates
- 1 tablespoon maple syrup or honey
- 1/2 teaspoon ground cinnamon
- 1/4 teaspoon ground nutmeg (optional)
- A pinch of ground ginger (optional)
- A dash of vanilla extract
- A dollop of Greek yogurt for topping (optional).

Method:

1. In a jar or container, combine rolled oats, milk, grated carrots, chopped nuts, raisins or chopped dates, maple syrup or honey, ground cinnamon, ground nutmeg (if using), ground ginger (if using), and vanilla extract. Mix well to combine all ingredients thoroughly.

2. Seal the jar or container and place it in the refrigerator. Let it refrigerate overnight or for at least 4 hours.

3. The next morning, give the oats a good stir. If the mixture is too thick, add a splash of milk and mix well.

4. Top your Carrot Cake Overnight Oats with a dollop of Greek yogurt for a creamy finish if desired.

5. Enjoy the flavors of carrot cake in your breakfast! This recipe offers a delightful blend of carrots, nuts, and spices reminiscent of carrot cake, providing a deliciously satisfying and nutritious morning meal. Adjust sweetness or add more spices to suit your taste.

Tiramisu Temptation Overnight Oats recipe

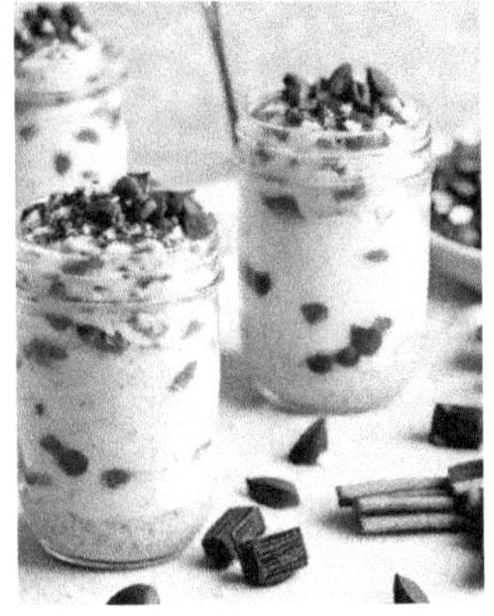

Try the Tiramisu Temptation Overnight Oats for a change in your breakfast routine. It's like having the flavors of a coffee-chocolate dessert, but in a healthier oatmeal form.

It's quick to prepare, and you'll wake up to a tasty, ready-to-eat breakfast that's a bit different from the usual oats. Plus, you can adjust the sweetness and coffee-chocolate flavors to your liking.

If you're a fan of the dessert or want to try something new for breakfast, these oats offer a fun and delicious twist to kickstart your day!

Prep Time: 5 minutes

Serving: 1

Ingredients:
- 1/2 cup rolled oats (old-fashioned oats)
- 1/2 cup milk (dairy or non-dairy)
- 1 tablespoon brewed coffee (cooled)
- 1 tablespoon cocoa powder
- 1 tablespoon maple syrup or honey
- 1/4 teaspoon vanilla extract
- A sprinkle of ground cinnamon (optional)
- A dollop of Greek yogurt for topping (optional for a more creamy taste)

- Chocolate shavings for garnish (optional)

Method:

1. In a jar or container, combine rolled oats, milk, brewed coffee, cocoa powder, maple syrup or honey, vanilla extract, and ground cinnamon if desired. Mix well to ensure all ingredients are thoroughly combined.

2. Seal the jar or container and place it in the refrigerator. Let it refrigerate overnight or for at least 4 hours.

3. The next morning, stir the oats thoroughly. If the mixture is too thick, add a splash of milk and mix well to reach your desired consistency.

4. Top your Tiramisu Temptation Overnight Oats with a dollop of Greek yogurt for a creamy touch, and garnish with chocolate shavings if desired.

Red Velvet Delight Overnight Oat recipe

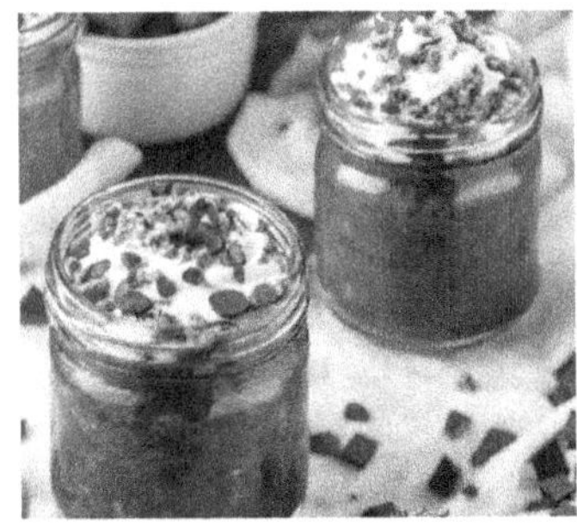

The Red Velvet Delight Overnight Oats offer a twist on the classic cake flavor in a convenient breakfast form. It's an easy-to-make recipe combining oats, cocoa powder, and a touch of sweetness, providing a tasty different flavor.

Prep Time: 5 minutes

Serving: 1

Ingredients:
- 1/2 cup rolled oats (old-fashioned oats)
- 1/2 cup milk (dairy or non-dairy)
- 1 tablespoon cocoa powder
- 1 tablespoon maple syrup or honey
- 1/4 teaspoon vanilla extract
- Red food coloring
- A dollop of Greek yogurt for topping (optional)
- Chocolate chips for garnish (optional)

Method:
1. In a jar or container, combine rolled oats, milk, cocoa powder, maple syrup or honey, vanilla extract, and a few drops of red food coloring if desired. Mix well to thoroughly combine all ingredients.

2. Seal the jar or container and place it in the refrigerator. Let it refrigerate overnight or for at least 4 hours.

3. The next morning, give the oats a good stir. If the mixture is too thick, add a splash of milk and mix well until you achieve your desired consistency.

4. Top your Red Velvet Delight Overnight Oats with a dollop of Greek yogurt for a creamy touch, and garnish with chocolate chips if desired.

Lemon Meringue Pie Overnight Oat recipe

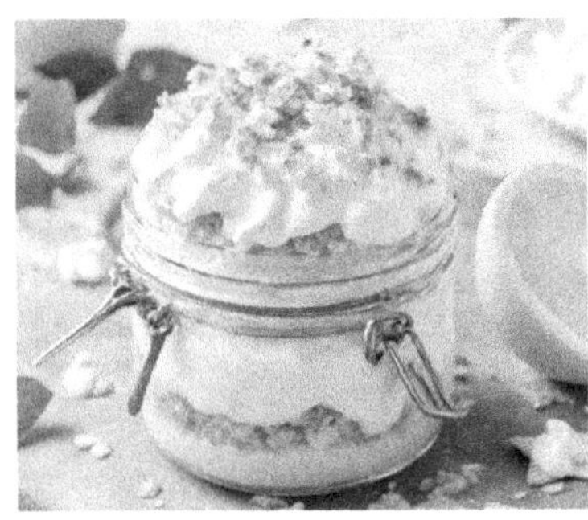

The Lemon Meringue Pie Overnight Oats offer a nutritious and delicious way to start your day, providing essential vitamins, fiber, and sustained energy to kickstart your day.

Prep Time: 5 minutes

Serving: 1

Ingredients:
- 1/2 cup rolled oats (old-fashioned oats)
- 1/2 cup milk (dairy or non-dairy)
- 2 tablespoons lemon juice (freshly squeezed)
- 1 tablespoon honey or maple syrup
- Zest of 1 lemon
- A dollop of Greek yogurt for topping (optional)
- Crushed graham crackers for garnish (optional)

Method:

1. In a jar or container, combine rolled oats, milk, lemon juice, honey or maple syrup, and the zest of one lemon. Stir well to mix all ingredients thoroughly.

2. Seal the jar or container and place it in the refrigerator. Let it refrigerate overnight or for at least 4 hours.

3. The next morning, stir the oats thoroughly. If the mixture is too thick, add a splash of milk and mix well to achieve your desired consistency.

4. Top your Lemon Meringue Pie Overnight Oats with a dollop of Greek yogurt for extra creaminess, and garnish with crushed graham crackers for a pie-like touch if desired.

Chapter 6: Savory and Unique Overnight Oats recipes

Savory Herb Overnight Oat recipe

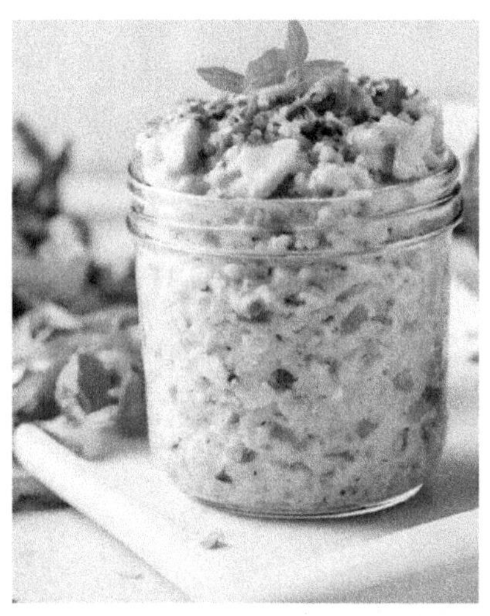

Savory Herb Overnight Oats give you a break from sweet breakfasts. They're all about adding fresh herbs like parsley or thyme to oats for a tasty, non-sweet twist in the morning. This is for those days you don't have a sweet tooth, when you are feeling the need for something spicy and healthy.

Prep Time: 5 minutes

Serving: 1

Ingredients:
- 1/2 cup rolled oats (old-fashioned oats)
- 1/2 cup chicken or vegetable broth (unsalted)
- 1 tablespoon chopped fresh herbs (such as parsley, chives, or thyme)
- 1/4 teaspoon garlic powder
- 1/4 teaspoon onion powder
- Salt and pepper to taste

- Optional toppings: chopped tomatoes, sliced avocado, or grated cheese

Method:

1. In a jar or container, combine rolled oats, chicken or vegetable broth, chopped fresh herbs, garlic powder, onion powder, salt, and pepper. Mix well to ensure all ingredients are thoroughly combined.

2. Seal the jar or container and place it in the refrigerator. Let it refrigerate overnight or for at least 6 hours.

3. The next morning, give the oats a good stir. If the mixture is too thick, add a splash of broth or water and mix well until you reach your desired consistency.

4. Serve your Savory Herb Overnight Oats topped with chopped tomatoes, sliced avocado, or grated cheese for extra flavor and texture, if desired.

Tomato Basil Overnight Oats

Recipe

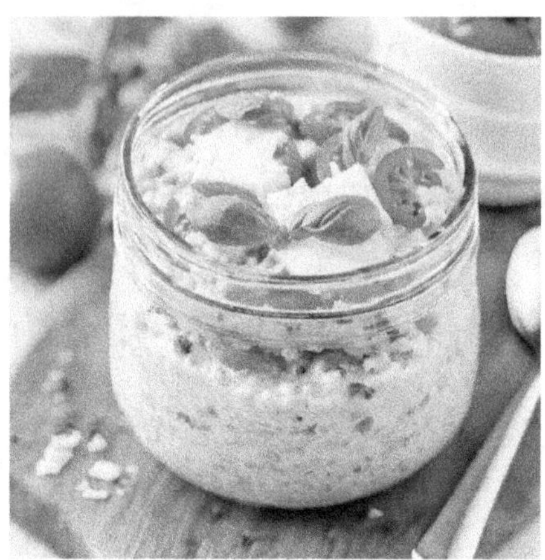

The Tomato Basil Overnight Oats recipe is a savory change from sweet oatmeal. It's made by mixing oats with tomato sauce or diced tomatoes, fresh basil, and some seasonings for a different breakfast taste.

Prep Time: 5 minutes

Serving: 1

Ingredients:
- 1/2 cup rolled oats
- 1/2 cup tomato sauce or diced tomatoes
- 1/4 cup vegetable or chicken broth
- 2-3 fresh basil leaves, chopped
- 1/4 teaspoon garlic powder
- Salt and pepper to taste
- Optional toppings: grated cheese, sliced cherry tomatoes, or a drizzle of olive oil

Method:
1. Combine rolled oats, tomato sauce or diced tomatoes, vegetable or chicken broth, chopped basil leaves, garlic powder, salt, and pepper in a jar or container.

2. Mix all ingredients thoroughly.

3. Seal the jar or container and refrigerate overnight or for at least 4 hours.

4. The next morning, give the oats a good stir. If it's too thick, add a bit more broth or water for your preferred consistency.

5. Serve your Tomato Basil Breakfast Oats with optional toppings like grated cheese, sliced cherry tomatoes, or a drizzle of olive oil.

Cheesy Spinach Overnight Oats recipe

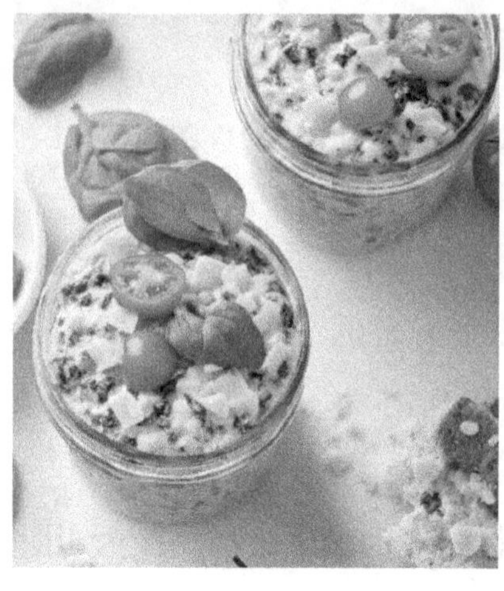

The Cheesy Spinach Overnight Oats combine the creamy richness of melted cheddar cheese with the nutritious goodness of spinach. The cheese adds a savory creaminess, while spinach brings in essential vitamins and minerals. Together, they create a tasty and nutrient-packed breakfast option.

Prep Time: 5 minutes

Serving: 1

Ingredients:
- 1/2 cup rolled oats
- 1/2 cup milk (dairy or non-dairy)
- 1/4 cup chopped spinach
- 1/4 cup shredded cheddar cheese
- Salt and pepper to taste
- Optional toppings: sliced cherry tomatoes, a sprinkle of more cheese, or a dash of hot sauce

Method:
1. In a jar or container, combine rolled oats, milk, chopped spinach, shredded cheddar cheese, salt, and pepper. Mix well to ensure all ingredients are thoroughly combined.
2. Seal the jar or container and place it in the refrigerator. Let it refrigerate overnight or for at least 4 hours.

3. The next morning, give the oats a good stir. If the mixture is too thick, add a splash of milk and mix well until you reach your desired consistency.

4. Serve your Cheesy Spinach Overnight Oats in a bowl and top them with optional toppings like sliced cherry tomatoes, extra cheese, or a dash of hot sauce for added flavor.

Mediterranean-Inspired Overnight Oat recipe

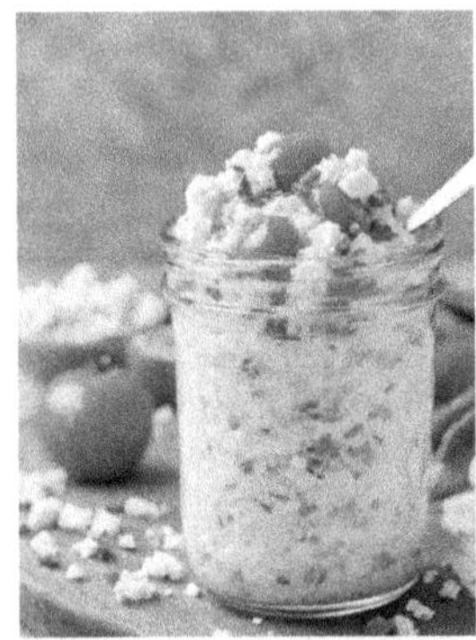

Enjoy the taste of the Mediterranean with these Overnight Oats. It's a mix of fresh veggies, herbs, and oats, bringing those vibrant Mediterranean flavors to your breakfast table..

Prep Time: 5 minutes

Serving: 1

Ingredients:
- 1/2 cup rolled oats
- 1/2 cup Greek yogurt
- 1/4 cup chopped cucumbers
- 1/4 cup chopped tomatoes
- 2 tablespoons chopped Kalamata olives
- 1 tablespoon chopped fresh parsley
- 1 tablespoon chopped fresh mint (optional)

- 1 tablespoon lemon juice
- Salt and pepper to taste
- Optional toppings: feta cheese, olive oil, or a sprinkle of za'atar seasoning

Method:

1. In a jar or container, layer rolled oats, Greek yogurt, chopped cucumbers, chopped tomatoes, chopped Kalamata olives, chopped fresh parsley, and chopped fresh mint if using.

2. Drizzle lemon juice over the ingredients.

3. Add a pinch of salt and pepper to taste.

4. Seal the jar or container and place it in the refrigerator. Let it refrigerate overnight or for at least 4 hours.

5. The next morning, give the oats a good stir to combine all the ingredients.

6. Serve your Mediterranean-Inspired Overnight Oats in a bowl and add optional toppings like feta cheese, a drizzle of olive oil, or a sprinkle of za'atar seasoning for extra flavor.

Creamy Mushroom Overnight Oats recipe

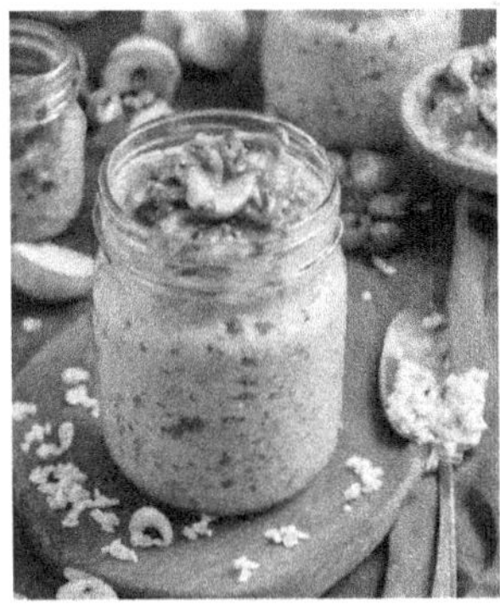

This creamy mushroom recipe gives that creamy savory taste packed with a blend of herbs and spice. It should be your go to recipe when you're in the mood for something that's both creamy and spicy.

Prep Time: 5 minutes

Cook Time: 5 minutes (the next morning)

Serving: 1

Ingredients:
- 1/2 cup rolled oats
- 1 cup vegetable or chicken broth
- 1/2 cup chopped mushrooms
- 2 tablespoons Greek yogurt or cream cheese
- 1 tablespoon chopped green onions or chives
- Salt and pepper to taste
- Optional toppings: sautéed mushrooms, a sprinkle of Parmesan cheese, or a dash of hot sauce

Method:

1. In a jar or container, combine rolled oats, vegetable or chicken broth, chopped mushrooms, Greek yogurt or cream cheese, chopped green onions or chives, salt, and pepper. Mix well to combine all ingredients thoroughly.

2. Seal the jar or container and place it in the refrigerator. Let it refrigerate overnight or for at least 4 hours.

3. The next morning, give the oats a good stir. If you prefer them warm, heat the oats in the microwave or on the stovetop until heated through.

4. Serve your Creamy Mushroom Overnight Oats in a bowl and top them with optional toppings like sautéed mushrooms, a sprinkle of Parmesan cheese, or a dash of hot sauce for added flavor.

Chapter 7: Dietary-Focused and Specialized Overnight Oat Recipes

Vegan-Friendly Overnight Oats Recipe

Mixed Berry Vegan Overnight Oats Recipe

Prep time: 5 mins

Serving: 1

Ingredients:
- 1/2 cup rolled oats
- 1/2 cup almond milk, coconut milk(or any plant-based milk)
- 1/4 cup mixed berries (strawberries, blueberries, raspberries)
- 1 tablespoon maple syrup or agave nectar
- 1 tablespoon chia seeds (optional)
- A handful of nuts or seeds for topping (optional)

Method:
1. In a jar or container, mix rolled oats, almond milk, mixed berries, maple syrup or agave nectar, and chia seeds (if using).
2. Stir well and ensure all ingredients are thoroughly combined.
3. Seal the jar or container and place it in the refrigerator overnight or for at least 4 hours.
4. The next morning, give the oats a good stir. If desired, top with a handful of nuts or seeds before serving.

Peanut Butter Banana Vegan Overnight Oats Recipe

Prep time: 5 mins

Serving: 1

Ingredients:
- 1/2 cup rolled oats
- 1/2 cup almond milk or coconut milk (or any plant-based milk)
- 1 ripe banana, mashed
- 2 tablespoons peanut butter (or any nut or seed butter)
- 1 tablespoon maple syrup or agave nectar (optional)
- A sprinkle of cinnamon (optional)
- Sliced banana and a drizzle of peanut butter for topping (optional)

Method:
1. In a jar or container, combine rolled oats, almond milk, mashed banana, peanut butter, maple syrup or agave nectar (if using), and cinnamon (if desired).
2. Mix well until all ingredients are thoroughly combined.
3. Seal the jar or container and refrigerate overnight or for at least 4 hours.
4. The next morning, stir the oats and top with sliced banana and a drizzle of peanut butter if desired before serving.

Apple Cinnamon Vegan Overnight Oats Recipe

Prep time : 5 mins

Serving: 1

Ingredients:
- 1/2 cup rolled oats
- 1/2 cup almond milk (or any plant-based milk)
- 1/2 apple, chopped
- 1 tablespoon maple syrup or agave nectar
- 1/2 teaspoon ground cinnamon
- A handful of chopped nuts for topping (optional)

Method:
1. In a jar or container, combine rolled oats, almond milk, chopped apple, maple syrup or agave nectar, and ground cinnamon.
2. Mix well and ensure all ingredients are thoroughly combined.
3. Seal the jar or container and refrigerate overnight or for at least 4 hours.
4. The next morning, give the oats a good stir. Top with a handful of chopped nuts before serving if desired.

Gluten-Free Overnight Oats recipes

Banana Nut Gluten-Free Overnight Oats Recipe

Prep time: 5 mins

Serving : 1

Ingredients:
- 1/2 cup gluten-free rolled oats
- 1/2 cup almond milk (or any preferred milk)
- 1 ripe banana, mashed
- 2 tablespoons chopped nuts (walnuts, almonds, or pecans)
- 1 tablespoon maple syrup or honey (optional)
- A sprinkle of cinnamon (optional)
- Sliced bananas and extra nuts for topping (optional)

Method:
1. In a jar or container, combine gluten-free rolled oats, almond milk, mashed banana, chopped nuts, maple syrup or honey (if using), and cinnamon (if desired).
2. Mix well until all ingredients are thoroughly combined.
3. Seal the jar or container and refrigerate overnight or for at least 4 hours.
4. The next morning, stir the oats and top with sliced bananas and extra nuts if desired before serving.

Blueberry Chia Seed Gluten-Free Overnight Oats Recipe

Prep time: 5 mins

Serving: 1

Ingredients:
- 1/2 cup gluten-free rolled oats
- 1/2 cup almond milk (or any preferred milk)
- 1/4 cup fresh or frozen blueberries
- 1 tablespoon chia seeds
- 1 tablespoon maple syrup or agave nectar (optional)
- A splash of vanilla extract (optional)
- Fresh blueberries for topping (optional)

Method:
1. In a jar or container, mix gluten-free rolled oats, almond milk, blueberries, chia seeds, maple syrup or agave nectar (if using), and vanilla extract (if desired).
2. Stir well until all ingredients are thoroughly combined.
3. Seal the jar or container and refrigerate overnight or for at least 4 hours.
4. The next morning, give the oats a good stir and top with fresh blueberries before serving if desired.

Pumpkin Pie Spice Gluten-Free Overnight Oats recipe

Prep time: 5 mins

Serving: 1

Ingredients:
- 1/2 cup gluten-free rolled oats
- 1/2 cup almond milk (or any preferred milk)
- 2 tablespoons pumpkin puree
- 1 tablespoon maple syrup or honey
- 1/2 teaspoon pumpkin pie spice (or a mix of cinnamon, nutmeg, and cloves)
- A handful of pecans or walnuts for topping (optional)

Method:
1. In a jar or container, combine gluten-free rolled oats, almond milk, pumpkin puree, maple syrup or honey, and pumpkin pie spice.
2. Mix well until thoroughly combined.
3. Seal the jar or container and refrigerate overnight or for at least 4 hours.
4. The next morning, stir the oats and top with a handful of pecans or walnuts if desired before serving.

Chocolate Banana Gluten-Free Overnight Oats recipe

Prep time: 5 mins

Serving: 1

Ingredients:
- 1/2 cup gluten-free rolled oats
- 1/2 cup almond milk (or any preferred milk)
- 1 ripe banana, mashed
- 1 tablespoon cocoa powder
- 1 tablespoon maple syrup or honey
- A handful of sliced bananas or chocolate chips for topping (optional)

Method:
1. In a jar or container, mix gluten-free rolled oats, almond milk, mashed banana, cocoa powder, and maple syrup or honey.
2. Stir well until thoroughly combined.
3. Seal the jar or container and refrigerate overnight or for at least 4 hours.
4. The next morning, give the oats a good stir and top with sliced bananas or chocolate chips if desired before serving.

These Gluten-Free Overnight Oats recipes offer flavorful variations perfect for those following a gluten-sensitive diet. Adjust sweetness or toppings based on personal preference.

Low-Sugar and Sugar-Free Overnight Oats recipes

Low-Sugar Cinnamon Apple Overnight Oats Recipe

Prep time: 5 mins

Serving: 1

Ingredients:
- 1/2 cup rolled oats
- 1/2 cup unsweetened almond milk (or any preferred milk)
- 1/2 apple, diced
- 1 tablespoon chopped walnuts or almonds
- 1/2 teaspoon ground cinnamon
- 1 tablespoon Greek yogurt (optional, for creaminess)
- Stevia, erythritol, or monk fruit sweetener to taste

Method:
1. In a jar or container, combine rolled oats, almond milk, diced apple, chopped nuts, ground cinnamon, Greek yogurt (if using), and your chosen sweetener.
2. Stir well until thoroughly combined.
3. Seal the jar or container and refrigerate overnight or for at least 4 hours.
4. The next morning, give the oats a good stir before serving.

Sugar-Free Vanilla Berry Overnight Oats Recipe

Prep time: 5 mins

Serving: 1

Ingredients:
- 1/2 cup rolled oats
- 1/2 cup unsweetened almond milk (or any preferred milk)
- 1/4 cup mixed berries (strawberries, blueberries, raspberries)
- 1/2 teaspoon vanilla extract
- 1 tablespoon chia seeds (optional, for added thickness)
- Stevia, erythritol, or monk fruit sweetener to taste

Method:
1. In a jar or container, mix rolled oats, almond milk, mixed berries, vanilla extract, chia seeds (if using), and your chosen sweetener.
2. Stir well until thoroughly combined.
3. Seal the jar or container and refrigerate overnight or for at least 4 hours.
4. The next morning, stir the oats before serving.

Coconut Almond Butter Overnight Oats Recipe

Prep time: 5 mins

Serving: 1

Ingredients:
- 1/2 cup rolled oats
- 1/2 cup unsweetened coconut milk (or any preferred milk)
- 1 tablespoon almond butter
- 1 tablespoon unsweetened shredded coconut
- 1 tablespoon sliced almonds
- Stevia, erythritol, or monk fruit sweetener to taste

Method:
1. In a jar or container, combine rolled oats, coconut milk, almond butter, shredded coconut, sliced almonds, and your chosen sweetener.
2. Mix well until thoroughly combined.
3. Seal the jar or container and refrigerate overnight or for at least 4 hours.
4. The next morning, give the oats a good stir before serving.

Lemon Blueberry Chia Seed Overnight Oats Recipe

Prep time: 5 mins

Serving: 1

Ingredients:
- 1/2 cup rolled oats
- 1/2 cup unsweetened almond milk (or any preferred milk)
- 1/4 cup fresh or frozen blueberries
- 1 tablespoon chia seeds
- 1 tablespoon lemon juice (from fresh lemon)
- Lemon zest (optional)
- Stevia, erythritol, or monk fruit sweetener to taste

Method:
1. In a jar or container, mix rolled oats, almond milk, blueberries, chia seeds, lemon juice, lemon zest (if using), and your chosen sweetener.
2. Stir well until thoroughly combined.
3. Seal the jar or container and refrigerate overnight or for at least 4 hours.
4. The next morning, stir the oats before serving.

These Low-Sugar and Sugar-Free Overnight Oats recipes provide flavorful options without added sugars, utilizing natural sweetness from ingredients while still remaining a delicious meal. Adjust the sweetness to your preference.

High-Protein Overnight Oats recipes

Protein-Packed Peanut Butter Banana Overnight Oats recipe

Prep time: 5 mins

Serving: 1

Ingredients:
- 1/2 cup rolled oats
- 1/2 cup Greek yogurt
- 1/2 cup unsweetened almond milk (or any preferred milk)
- 1 ripe banana, mashed
- 2 tablespoons peanut butter (or any nut or seed butter)
- 1 tablespoon chia seeds
- 1 tablespoon honey or maple syrup (optional)
- Optional toppings: sliced banana, chopped nuts

Method:
1. In a jar or container, mix rolled oats, Greek yogurt, almond milk, mashed banana, peanut butter, chia seeds, and honey or maple syrup if using.
2. Stir well until thoroughly combined.
3. Seal the jar or container and refrigerate overnight or for at least 4 hours.
4. The next morning, stir the oats and top with sliced banana and chopped nuts if desired before serving.

High-Protein Chocolate Almond Overnight Oats Recipe

Prep time: 5 mins

Serving: 1

Ingredients:
- 1/2 cup rolled oats
- 1/2 cup unsweetened almond milk (or any preferred milk)
- 1/2 cup plain or chocolate-flavored protein powder
- 1 tablespoon cocoa powder (unsweetened)
- 1 tablespoon almond butter
- 1 tablespoon chia seeds
- Stevia, erythritol, or monk fruit sweetener to taste
- Optional toppings: sliced almonds, dark chocolate shavings

Method:
1. In a jar or container, combine rolled oats, almond milk, protein powder, cocoa powder, almond butter, chia seeds, and your chosen sweetener.
2. Mix well until thoroughly combined.
3. Seal the jar or container and refrigerate overnight or for at least 4 hours.
4. The next morning, stir the oats and top with sliced almonds and dark chocolate shavings if desired before serving.

Berry Protein Blast Overnight Oats Recipe

Prep time: 5 mins

Serving: 1

Ingredients:
- 1/2 cup rolled oats
- 1/2 cup Greek yogurt
- 1/2 cup unsweetened almond milk (or any preferred milk)
- 1/4 cup mixed berries (strawberries, blueberries, raspberries)
- 2 tablespoons vanilla protein powder
- 1 tablespoon chia seeds
- Stevia, erythritol, or monk fruit sweetener to taste
- Optional toppings: additional berries, sliced almonds

Method:
1. In a jar or container, mix rolled oats, Greek yogurt, almond milk, mixed berries, protein powder, chia seeds, and your chosen sweetener.
2. Stir well until thoroughly combined.
3. Seal the jar or container and refrigerate overnight or for at least 4 hours.
4. The next morning, give the oats a good stir and top with additional berries and sliced almonds if desired before serving.

Coconut Vanilla Protein Overnight Oats Recipe

Prep time: 5 mins

Serving: 1

Ingredients:
- 1/2 cup rolled oats
- 1/2 cup unsweetened coconut milk (or any preferred milk)
- 1/2 cup Greek yogurt
- 2 tablespoons vanilla protein powder
- 1 tablespoon shredded coconut (unsweetened)
- 1 tablespoon chia seeds
- Stevia, erythritol, or monk fruit sweetener to taste
- Optional toppings: sliced bananas, toasted coconut flakes

Method:
1. In a jar or container, combine rolled oats, coconut milk, Greek yogurt, protein powder, shredded coconut, chia seeds, and your chosen sweetener.
2. Mix well until thoroughly combined.
3. Seal the jar or container and refrigerate overnight or for at least 4 hours.
4. The next morning, stir the oats and top with sliced bananas and toasted coconut flakes if desired before serving.

These High-Protein Overnight Oats recipes are packed with protein-rich ingredients like Greek yogurt, protein powder, chia seeds, and nuts, providing a delicious and satisfying breakfast. Adjust sweetness or toppings according to your taste preferences.

Chapter 8: Customizing Your Overnight Oats

Tips for Customizing Recipes

Here's how you can make Overnight Oats your own way:

1. Pick Your Oats: Choose what type of oats you like - there are different kinds like rolled oats or quick oats. Add some milk or yogurt as your starting liquid.

2. Sweeten It Up: If you want your oats sweet, you can add a little honey, maple syrup, or mashed fruits like bananas or berries.

3. Add Fun Stuff: Mix in things you like - fruits such as berries, apples, or bananas; nuts or seeds like almonds, chia seeds, or pumpkin seeds; or even some yummy spices like cinnamon or vanilla.

4. Boost It with Protein: If you want more protein, you can put in some protein powder, Greek yogurt, or cottage cheese.

5.Make It Fancy: Put toppings on it! Add things like more fruit slices, nuts, seeds, coconut flakes, or even a few chocolate chips.

6. Change the Texture: You can make it smoother by blending some parts or layering it with fruit or yogurt. Play around to see what you like!

7. Wait Time: Let your oats sit in the fridge overnight or for a few hours until they get soft. If you like them softer, leave them longer. If you prefer them a bit chewy, less time is okay.

By mixing and matching these steps, you can create your own unique Overnight Oats every morning. Have fun trying out different combinations to make your breakfast just the way you like it!

Personalizing Flavors and Textures

Personalizing flavors and textures in your Overnight Oats recipes, can be a fun way to tailor your breakfast to your liking. Here are some simple ways to do it:

1. Flavor Enhancements:
Fruit Infusions: Experiment with various fruits - fresh, frozen, or dried. Mash or blend fruits like bananas, strawberries, or blueberries and mix them in for added natural sweetness and flavor.

Spice It Up: Add spices such as cinnamon, nutmeg, or cardamom to create warm and aromatic flavors in your oats. A little goes a long way!

Extracts and Essences: Vanilla, almond, or citrus extracts can add depth and aroma. A few drops can make a significant difference.

2.Texture Tweaks:
Crunchy Additions: Incorporate nuts (like almonds, walnuts, or pecans), seeds (chia seeds, flaxseeds, pumpkin seeds), or granola for a crunchy texture.

Creaminess Boost: Mix in Greek yogurt, coconut cream, or nut butter to add creaminess and richness to your oats.

Fruit Layers: Layer your oats with sliced fruits or fruit preserves to create a layered, textured experience.

3. Customizing Sweetness:

Natural Sweeteners: Use honey, maple syrup, mashed ripe bananas, or applesauce for sweetness without relying on refined sugars.

Stevia or Monk Fruit: If you prefer a calorie-free option, these natural sweeteners can add sweetness without impacting blood sugar levels.

4.Protein-Packed Options:

Protein Sources: Incorporate protein powder, Greek yogurt, cottage cheese, or almond butter to increase the protein content for a more satisfying meal.

5. Soaking Time Variations:

Texture Preference: Adjust the soaking time based on your preferred oat texture. Longer soaking creates softer oats, while shorter soaking retains more chewiness.

6. Toppings and Finishes:

 Custom Toppings: Have fun with toppings! Consider fresh fruit slices, dried coconut, dark chocolate chips, or a sprinkle of your favorite seeds for added variety and appeal.

By experimenting with these ideas, you can create a wide array of flavors and textures in your Overnight Oats to suit your taste preferences and make your breakfasts more enjoyable!

Make-Ahead and Storage Tips

1. Prepare in Advance:
   - Overnight Oats are meant to be made ahead! Prepare them the night before or several hours before you plan to eat them to allow time for the oats to soften and refrigerate up the flavors.

2. Batch Preparation:
   - Make a batch of multiple servings at once to have breakfast ready for a few days. Store them in individual jars or containers for convenience.

3. Proper Storage:
   - Use airtight containers or jars with lids to store Overnight Oats in the refrigerator. This prevents air exposure and helps maintain freshness.

4. Refrigeration Time:
   - Let your prepared Overnight Oats sit in the refrigerator for at least 4 hours or ideally overnight. This allows the oats to absorb the liquid and flavors properly.

5. Customization After Refrigeration:
   - Add fresh toppings or garnishes right before serving rather than storing them with the oats. This keeps toppings like fruits or nuts fresher and crunchier, except the recipe calls for infusion or soaking.

6. Storage Duration:

- Overnight Oats can typically be stored in the refrigerator for up to 3-4 days. However, toppings and fruits may lose their freshness after a day or two.

7. Texture Check:

- Give the oats a good stir before eating. If the mixture seems too thick, you can add a splash of milk or yogurt to loosen it up.

8. Individual Portions:

- If preparing multiple servings, consider using jars or containers with measurements marked on them. This way, you can easily grab the right portion without needing to measure every time.

9. Freezing Option (Optional):

- While Overnight Oats are typically stored in the fridge, you can experiment with freezing smaller portions in airtight containers. Thaw them in the refrigerator overnight before consuming.

10.Experiment with Variations:

- Try different flavor combinations and ingredients to keep your breakfast exciting and to find out which combinations store best for your preferences.

By following these tips, you can efficiently prepare, store, and enjoy your Overnight Oats without any hassle each day!

Overnight Oats are a convenient breakfast choice you can prepare ahead of time. You mix oats with different things like milk, fruits, nuts, and spices to make tasty combinations. They're good because you can make them the night before and keep them in the fridge for a few days.

These oats are healthy and provide energy for the day. You can make them the way you like by trying different ingredients and adjusting how long you refrigerate them. They're a flexible breakfast that you can make your own!.